NUTRITION AND EXERCISE

FOR

WEIGHT LOSS

The Ultimate Handbook for Healthy Living

DR. J. K. EVANS

TABLE OF CONTENT

Overview of Weight Loss Goals

Many people who wish to get healthier, look better, or be more fit have weight loss as one of their common goals. But not everyone has the same objectives when it comes to losing weight, and individuals may have different drives, expectations, and justifications. Therefore, before you embark on your path, it's critical to have a concise and realistic assessment of your weight loss goals.

Finding your current weight and body mass index (BMI), which is a measurement of your body fat based on your height and weight, is one of the first steps in creating a weight loss plan. To determine your BMI, use internet calculators or speak with your physician. A BMI of 18.5 to 24.9 is considered healthy, while a BMI of 25 or higher denotes overweight, and a BMI of 30 or above suggests obesity. You can evaluate your health risks and determine how much weight loss is necessary to reach a healthy weight by knowing your BMI.

Determining your motives and reasons for wanting to lose weight is a necessary step in creating your weight reduction objectives. Several typical causes of weight loss include:

- To lower the chance of developing chronic illnesses like diabetes, heart disease, stroke, and some types of cancer.

- To enhance life quality, including increased vitality, mobility, self-assurance, and self-worth.

- To fulfill a desire, either personal or professional, such getting a certain size, competing in a sport or event, or developing in a career.

- To improve one's looks, such as by appearing more appealing, youthful, or trim.

Make sure your motivations are clear, significant, and constructive for you, whatever they may be. Strong motivation can support you in maintaining commitment and focus on your weight loss program.

Making your weight reduction goals SMART—Specific, Measurable, Achievable, Relevant, and Time-bound—is the last stage in creating your goals. Compared to ambiguous or unattainable goals, SMART goals are more practical and productive. A SMART goal might be, for instance, "I want to lose 10 kg in 6 months by following a balanced diet and exercising for 30 minutes a day, five times a week," as opposed to just "I want to lose weight." With the use of SMART goals, you may monitor your development, recognize your successes, and modify your strategy as necessary.

Importance of Nutrition and Exercise

The term "nutrition" describes the foods and beverages you eat and how they impact your body's metabolism and other processes. Because nutrition affects both how much energy you use and how many calories you consume, it is essential for weight loss. You must generate a calorie deficit—that is, burn more calories than you take in—in order to lose weight. Eating less, eating better, or doing both will help you reach your goal.

Reducing your portion sizes, limiting your snacking, and avoiding overeating are all part of eating less. Eating a healthier diet entail selecting items that are high in protein, fiber, vitamins, and minerals and low in calories, fat, sugar, and salt. Fruits, vegetables, whole grains, lean meats, low-fat dairy, nuts, seeds, and legumes are a few types of healthful foods. You may increase your metabolism, feel fuller for longer, and avoid cravings by eating these items.

Exercise is the term used to describe your physical activities and how they impact your body's metabolism and functions. Exercise is essential for weight loss because it affects both the amount of muscle you gain and the number of calories you burn. You must increase your physical activity—that is, move more, exercise more, or do both—if you want to reduce weight.

Increasing your daily activities, such as walking, using the stairs, taking care of home tasks, or playing with your children, is the equivalent of moving more. Increasing your physical activity level entails participating in regimented routines like aerobic, strength, or flexibility training. You may increase your muscle mass, burn calories, and strengthen your heart and muscles by doing these workouts.

Exercise and proper nutrition are crucial for losing weight, but they also improve your general health in other ways. Exercise and proper diet can benefit you:

Enhance your mental and emotional well-being by releasing endorphins, serotonin, and dopamine—neurotransmitters that promote contentment, calmness, and motivation.

- Because they lower blood pressure, cholesterol, blood sugar, and inflammatory levels, they can help lessen your chance of developing chronic diseases like diabetes, heart disease, stroke, and some malignancies.

- Improve your appearance by making you appear younger, thinner, and more alluring by improving your skin, hair, nails, and body form.

- Increasing your self-esteem and confidence will help you feel good about yourself and your accomplishments.

Chapter 1:

Understanding Weight Loss

Body Composition and Metabolism

Two major factors that influence your weight reduction outcomes are your body composition and metabolism. The percentage of fat, muscle, bone, and water in your body is known as your body composition, and the pace at which your body burns calories for energy is known as your metabolism. Gaining an understanding of these elements can help you reach your objectives and optimize your weight loss approach.

Your body composition affects how many calories you burn and how much you need, which makes it crucial for weight loss. Numerous factors, including age, gender, genetics, and lifestyle, affect your body composition. Your metabolism will typically increase and you will burn more calories even when at rest if you have greater muscle mass. On the other hand, even while you're at rest, your metabolism slows down and you burn less calories the more fat you have.

As a result, you must improve your muscle mass and decrease your body fat proportion in order to lose weight. A balanced diet that includes adequate amounts of protein, carbs, and healthy fats along with vitamins, minerals, and water will help you do this.

In particular, protein is necessary for both keeping and growing muscle as well as for keeping you full and content. Fats and carbohydrates are also necessary for energy production and the maintenance of certain body processes.

You must follow a diet in addition to getting regular exercise, which should include both aerobic and anaerobic activities. Running, swimming, cycling, and dancing are examples of aerobic exercises that are good for burning fat and calories while also strengthening your heart and lungs. Anaerobic workouts, like weightlifting, resistance training, or high-intensity interval training, are good for increasing muscle mass and strength while also improving hormone balance and metabolism.

Because metabolism controls how well your body uses the calories you eat and burn, it is crucial for weight loss. Your age, gender, lifestyle, and genetics all affect your metabolism. In general, your metabolism increases with age, meaning that even while you're at rest, you burn more calories. On the other hand, as you age, your metabolism decreases and you burn less calories overall, even while you're at rest.

As a result, you must consume fewer calories and raise your metabolic rate in order to lose weight.

This can be accomplished by eating a balanced diet that is high in fiber, protein, and complex carbohydrates—all of which can help you feel fuller for longer and stop overeating—and that offers just the right number of calories. Foods heavy in calories, fat, sugar, and salt should also be avoided since they might slow down metabolism and result in weight gain.

You must follow a diet in addition to getting regular exercise, which should include both aerobic and anaerobic activities. Anaerobic activities can help you gain muscle and speed up your metabolism, while aerobic exercises can help you burn fat and calories. Along with mixing up your workouts and intensities, you can keep your body from becoming too accustomed to one particular pattern and hitting a plateau. You should also incorporate some metabolism-boosting activities, including drinking coffee, green tea, or water, eating spicy foods, or taking cold baths.

Factors Influencing Weight Loss

Losing weight is a difficult process with many facets and internal and environmental variables that can impact your outcome. While some of these factors—like your food, exercise routine, and lifestyle choices—are under your control, other factors—like your genetics, age, gender, and underlying medical conditions—are not.

You may maximize your strategy and accomplish your objectives by being aware of how these variables affect your weight reduction.

Several internal factors can impact your ability to lose weight, including:

- Genetics: Your metabolism, appetite, distribution of body fat, and reaction to certain meals and activities can all be influenced by your genes. It's possible that some people are genetically predisposed to gaining or losing weight more quickly than others, or to storing fat in particular body parts. Nevertheless, you can still lose weight by adhering to a healthy, balanced diet and exercise regimen that is appropriate for your body type and needs. Genetics are not destiny.

- Hormones: By controlling your hunger, satiety, energy, mood, and stress levels, hormones can have an impact on your ability to lose weight. Leptin, ghrelin, insulin, and cortisol are some examples of hormones that, depending on their function and balance, can either encourage or impede weight loss. Hormonal imbalances can complicate weight loss and arise from a variety of causes, including aging, pregnancy, menopause, stress, sleep deprivation, and medical diseases. Consequently, it's critical to follow a healthy lifestyle that can assist in naturally balancing your hormones and to speak with your doctor if you think you may have a hormonal problem.

- Psychology: Your motivation, attitude, behavior, and emotions are all influenced by your psychology, which might have an impact on your weight reduction. While some psychological issues, like melancholy, anxiety, low self-esteem, and emotional eating, might impede weight loss, others, including self-efficacy, optimism, resilience, and social support, can help you lose weight. Consequently, it's critical to deal with any psychological problems that might be preventing you from losing weight and, if necessary, to get professional assistance. Together with avoiding self-criticism and having irrational expectations, you should also work on having a good outlook and a healthy connection with food and your body.

The following are a few outside variables that may affect your weight loss:

- Environment: Your surroundings can either make it easier or harder for you to lose weight by giving you access to opportunities for physical activity and wholesome eating. Availability, cost, convenience, and social norms are examples of environmental factors that, depending on your location, culture, and socioeconomic level, can either help or hinder your weight loss efforts. As a result, it's critical to understand how your surroundings affect your ability to lose weight and to act sensibly given the conditions. Additionally, you want to make an effort to establish a friendly and encouraging environment for your weight reduction. Some examples of this include putting nutritious food in your kitchen, signing up for a fitness class or gym, or finding a weight loss coach or partner.

- Lifestyle: Your everyday routines and habits have the power to either facilitate or impede weight loss, thus they can have an impact on how much weight you lose. The quality, quantity, and frequency of some lifestyle factors, like nutrition, exercise, sleep, stress, and smoking, can have a big effect on how much weight you lose. In order to support your weight reduction, it is crucial to maintain a healthy, balanced lifestyle. You should also try to reduce or prevent any bad habits that could interfere with your weight loss efforts. Aside from trying to alter your lifestyle in a realistic and sustainable way, you should also keep track of your efforts and outcomes.

Chapter 2:
Nutrition Fundamentals

Macronutrients: Carbohydrates, Proteins, Fats

The primary ingredients in meals that give the body energy and necessary nutrition are called macronutrients. They are separated into three groups: lipids, proteins, and carbs. Every macronutrient performs a distinct purpose in the body and affects weight reduction in a unique way. Gaining knowledge about the functions of macronutrients will help you adjust your diet and reach your weight loss objectives.

The body uses carbohydrates as its main energy source, particularly for the muscles and brain. They are made up of glucose molecules that are broken down from sugar molecules and either consumed immediately or stored as glycogen. There are two categories of carbohydrates: simple and complicated. Simple carbs allow blood sugar levels to rise and fall quickly after digestion and are present in meals including fruits, milk, honey, and refined sugar. Whole grains, beans, vegetables, and nuts are examples of diets high in complex carbs. These foods digest slowly and release glucose gradually over time.

Because they offer energy and satiety and because they can affect the hormones that control appetite and metabolism, carbohydrates are crucial for weight loss. But not all carbohydrates are created equal, and some may help or hinder weight loss more than others. Because complex carbs contain a lot of fiber, which can help you feel fuller for longer, lower your cholesterol, and enhance the health of your digestive system, they are generally better for weight reduction. Conversely, simple carbs are more likely to make you gain weight since they are high in calories, low in nutrients, and can raise insulin and blood sugar levels, which can result in the accumulation of fat and an increase in appetite.

Because proteins are made up of amino acids, which are needed to produce and repair different tissues like muscles, bones, skin, hair, and nails, they are known as the building blocks of the body. Furthermore, they have a role in a variety of biochemical activities, including immune system activity, hormone synthesis, and enzyme manufacturing. Plant sources like soy, beans, lentils, and quinoa, as well as animal ones like meat, eggs, dairy, and fish, are good sources of protein.

Because they promote satiety, thermogenesis, and muscle preservation, proteins are crucial for weight loss. Proteins have the ability to satiate you, allowing you to eat less calories and feel fuller for longer.

Because proteins need more energy to digest and metabolize than fats or carbs, thermogenesis implies that eating proteins can raise your metabolic rate and burn more calories. Proteins can help you retain or grow your lean body mass, which can speed up your metabolism and stop you from losing muscle mass when losing weight. This is known as muscle preservation.

Since fats have nine calories per gram, compared to four for proteins or carbs, fats are the body's most concentrated source of energy. They are made up of three different kinds of fatty acids: trans, unsaturated, and saturated. Foods like butter, cheese, cream, and fatty meats contain saturated fats, which are solid at room temperature. Nuts, seeds, avocados, olive oil, and other foods that are liquid at room temperature include unsaturated fats. Trans fats are produced artificially by hydrogenating unsaturated fats and can be found in foods like margarine, baked products, and fried foods.

Because they offer satiety, energy, and vital nutrients like omega-3 and omega-6 fatty acids—which are involved in a number of processes like blood coagulation, inflammation, and brain development—fats are crucial for weight loss. But not all fats are created equal, and some may help or hinder weight loss more than others. Due to their high content of monounsaturated and polyunsaturated fatty acids, which can lower cholesterol, enhance cardiovascular health, and lessen the risk of diabetes, unsaturated fats are generally better for weight loss. Conversely, because they are high in calories and poor in nutrients, saturated and trans fats have the potential to induce inflammation, raise cholesterol, and reduce insulin sensitivity, all of which increase the likelihood of weight gain.

Micronutrients: Vitamins and Minerals

The body requires micronutrients, which are tiny but vital nutrients, in trace amounts to carry out a number of processes, including metabolism, growth, development, and immunity. Minerals and vitamins make up the two groups into which they fall. The two types of chemical molecules known as vitamins are fat-soluble and water-soluble. Water-soluble vitamins, such B-complex vitamins and vitamin C, dissolve in water and are eliminated through urine; therefore, they must be continuously supplied. Vitamins A, D, E, and K are fat-soluble vitamins that are stored in fat cells and the liver. If ingested in excess, they can build up to hazardous levels. There are two categories of inorganic elements known as minerals: macro minerals and trace minerals. Whereas trace minerals like iron, zinc, iodine, and selenium are needed in lesser amounts, macro minerals like calcium, magnesium, sodium, and potassium are needed in greater quantities.

Because they promote a number of processes and functions related to energy production, hunger regulation, fat burning, muscle growth, and water balance, micronutrients are crucial for weight loss. Not all micronutrients, though, have the same effects on weight loss; in fact, some may even be counterproductive. Given their beneficial impacts on weight loss, the following micronutrients are generally better for weight loss:

- Vitamin C: This water-soluble vitamin supports the immune system, synthesizes collagen, and functions as an antioxidant. By increasing fat oxidation, lowering inflammation, and raising insulin sensitivity, vitamin C can aid in weight loss. Foods high in vitamin C include broccoli, kiwis, peppers, berries, and citrus fruits.

- Vitamin D: A fat-soluble vitamin that regulates calcium, builds bones, and functions as a hormone. By decreasing the synthesis of cortisol, a hormone that increases hunger and encourages fat storage, and increasing the production of leptin, a hormone that suppresses appetite and signals satiety, vitamin D can aid in weight loss. Supplements, fortified meals, and sun exposure are good sources of vitamin D.

- Vitamin B12: This water-soluble vitamin functions as a coenzyme, nerve guard, and synthesis of DNA. By enhancing the metabolism of proteins, lipids, and carbs as well as elevating mood and energy levels, vitamin B12 can aid in weight loss.

Foods including meat, eggs, dairy products, fish, and shellfish all contain vitamin B12, as do supplements.

- Iron: An essential trace mineral, iron serves as an oxygen carrier, an enzyme cofactor, and a component of hemoglobin. By increasing aerobic capacity and endurance as well as the flow of oxygen and nutrients to the muscles and organs, iron can aid in weight loss. Foods high in iron include red meat, chicken, fish, beans, spinach, fortified cereals, and spinach supplements.

- Zinc: This trace mineral strengthens the immune system, promotes wound healing, and is an antioxidant. Zinc increases thermogenesis and fat burning and regulates hunger-controlling hormones like ghrelin and leptin to aid in weight loss. Foods including oysters, meat, chicken, nuts, seeds, dairy products, and supplements all contain zinc.

- Magnesium: A macro mineral, magnesium relaxes muscles, stabilizes nerves, and activates enzymes. Magnesium can aid in weight reduction by lowering stress and anxiety, which can lead to emotional eating and cravings, and by enhancing the quantity and quality of sleep, which can influence the hormones that control appetite and metabolism. Foods like dark chocolate, bananas, avocados, nuts, seeds, leafy greens, and supplements all contain magnesium.

Calories and Energy Balance

The ideas of calories and energy balance are fundamental to comprehending and attaining weight loss. Calories are a unit of measurement for energy that the body utilizes for a variety of processes and activities. They are obtained from food. The link between the number of calories the body uses and the number of calories it consumes is known as energy balance. You may maximize your diet and exercise regimen and reach your weight loss objectives by being aware of how calories and energy balance function.

Because they affect how much weight you acquire or lose over time, calories are crucial for weight loss. You must achieve a negative energy balance, or burn more calories than you take in, in order to lose weight. Either burning more calories or consuming less calories will do this. The number of calories you need to burn and eat relies on a number of variables, including your age, gender, height, weight, degree of exercise, and objective of losing weight. To determine your desired daily caloric deficit, you can speak with your doctor or use internet calculators.

But not all calories are created equal, and some may be more helpful or harmful to losing weight than others. In general, since calories have an impact on your hunger, satiety, metabolism, and hormones, the kind and timing of your calorie intake can determine how much weight you lose.

Calories from fat, sugar, and alcohol, on the other hand, might make you feel hungry sooner and slow down your metabolism. For instance, calories from protein, fiber, and complex carbs can help you feel fuller for longer and increase your metabolism. Similar to this, consuming calories in the morning can provide you energy for the day and help you avoid overindulging later, whereas consuming calories at night can disrupt your sleep, cause digestive problems, and encourage the storage of fat.

Because it controls how your body reacts to the calories you ingest and burn, energy balance is crucial for weight loss. A negative energy balance is necessary for weight loss, but it shouldn't be too low because this might have detrimental effects on both your health and your ability to lose weight. Your body may go into starvation mode, which lowers metabolism, increases appetite, preserves fat reserves, and breaks down muscular tissue for energy, if your energy balance is too negative. This may increase the difficulty and unsustainable nature of weight reduction, increase the risk of weight gain, and cause health issues.

As a result, maintaining a modest and steady negative energy balance—that is, burning more calories than you take in—is necessary for weight loss. Without endangering your health and metabolism, you can safely and steadily lose weight with the support of a moderately and consistently negative energy balance.

It is often advised to aim for a 500 calorie daily negative energy balance, which can lead to 0.5 kg of weekly weight loss. You can change your calorie intake and expenditure in accordance with your own circumstances and tastes, though.

Chapter 3:
Designing a Healthy Eating Plan
Portion Control and Serving Sizes

Two related ideas that can assist you in controlling your calorie intake and reaching your weight loss objectives are portion control and serving sizes. Serving size is the normal amount of food that is advised by nutrition experts or product labels, whereas portion control is the quantity of food that you choose to eat at a specific moment. You may optimize your diet and prevent overeating by being aware of how serving sizes and portion management operate.

Portion control is crucial for weight loss because it can help you burn more calories than you take in by limiting your calorie intake and establishing a negative energy balance. You must be conscious of how much food you are eating and how it compares to the suggested serving size in order to practice portion control. To measure your portions, you can use a variety of tools, including scales, measuring cups, spoons, and your hand. Additionally, you can utilize visual clues. For example, you can compare your portions to everyday objects like a computer mouse, a deck of cards, or a tennis ball.

Because it can help you balance your macronutrients—carbs, proteins, and fats—and plan your meals and snacks, serving size is crucial for weight loss. You can utilize applications or internet resources to find the portion size of cooked or fresh food, or you can read the nutrition data label on packaged items. Another option is to divide your meal into four halves using the plate technique, which is as easy as dividing it into half for veggies, 1/4 for lean protein, and 1/4 for whole grains or starchy vegetables. On the side, you can also include a tiny amount of cheese and fruit.

Serving sizes and portion sizes are important for weight reduction, but they are not the same and can change based on a number of variables, including your age, gender, height, weight, degree of exercise, and weight loss objective. Consequently, you ought to modify your portions in accordance with your own requirements and tastes rather than depending just on the serving size. The timing and quality of your meals should also be taken into account as they may have an impact on your ability to lose weight. For instance, to help you feel fuller for longer and speed up your metabolism, choose portions that are high in fiber, protein, and complex carbs and low in calories, fat, sugar, and salt. In addition, eating smaller, more frequent meals throughout the day is preferable than eating bigger, less frequent ones since it can help you control your insulin and blood sugar levels, as well as curb cravings and hunger.

Meal Planning Strategies

Planning your meals can help you manage your calorie intake, balance your macronutrients, and avoid overindulging and cravings—all of which are important weight loss strategies. Meal planning is deciding what, when, and how much to eat for each meal and snack, as well as preparing or buying the necessary foods and components. In addition to lowering your stress levels and saving money and time, meal planning can also enhance your wellbeing. The following guidelines and actions will help you plan meals effectively for weight loss:

- Establish your daily calorie budget and weight loss objective: Prior to beginning meal planning, ascertain your daily calorie budget and weight loss objective. To determine your desired daily caloric deficit, you can speak with your doctor or use internet calculators. It is often advised to aim for a 500 calorie daily negative energy balance, which can lead to 0.5 kg of weekly weight loss. You can change your calorie intake and expenditure in accordance with your own circumstances and tastes, though.

- Select the frequency and timing of your meals: The next step is to determine the number of meals and snacks you will have each day, as well as the times of day.

As long as you keep within your calorie budget and achieve a negative energy balance, you can choose a meal frequency and timing that works for your appetite, schedule, and lifestyle. Eating three main meals and one or two snacks per day, separated by three to four hours, is a popular alternative. Additionally, eating at regular, consistent times—as well as avoiding eating too late at night—will help you better control your hunger, metabolism, and quality of sleep.

- Plan your menu and recipes: Next, you must consider your macronutrient balance and calorie budget when creating your menu and recipes for each meal and snack. Foods heavy in calories, fat, sugar, and salt, including processed, fried, or fast food, should be avoided or consumed in moderation. Instead, you should try to eat a range of foods from different food groups, such as fruits, vegetables, whole grains, lean proteins, healthy fats, and low-fat dairy. Additionally, you want to make an effort to incorporate nutritious culinary techniques like baking, grilling, steaming, or roasting into your meals and snacks to make them tasty, colorful, and filling. You can make your own recipes based on your tastes and creativity or use internet resources or apps to locate delicious and nutritious recipes that meet your macronutrient and calorie goals.

- Purchase and prepare food: The last step is to shop, prepare, and store your food for your scheduled meals and snacks in the pantry, refrigerator, or freezer, depending on how long they will last and how you plan to use it. When you visit the market or grocery store, you should develop a shopping list based on your meal and dishes, and follow it. Additionally, you should try to avoid shopping when you're hungry because this increases the likelihood that you'll purchase unneeded or harmful food. Additionally, you want to make an effort to prepare your meals ahead of time, ideally the night before or over the weekend, and split them into bags or containers so that you can quickly grab and go as needed. Additionally, you can measure your serving sizes and amounts using equipment like measuring cups, spoons, scales, or your hand. Label each item with the name, date, and nutritional facts, including calories and macronutrients.

Reading Food Labels

Knowing how to read food labels can help you make healthy, educated decisions about the foods and beverages you eat and drink, which is a useful skill for weight loss. Food labels give you a wealth of information about a product, including ingredients, nutrition statistics, serving sizes, and health claims. You can use this information to evaluate goods and choose the ones that best fit your needs and weight loss objectives. To help you understand food labels and lose weight, consider the following advice and steps:

Take a look at the components list. It lists every ingredient used to create the product in descending weight order. You can determine the quality and quantity of the contents by looking at the ingredients list. You may also limit or stay away from ingredients like oils, butter, syrup, and sodium that are rich in calories, fat, sugar, and salt. Additionally, you should check for the presence of artificial flavors, colors, and preservatives, as they can interfere with your ability to lose weight and improve your health. Selecting items with fewer, simpler ingredients and those created from whole, natural foods like fruits, vegetables, grains, nuts, and seeds is something you should strive for.

- Examine the panel with dietary facts: The product's calories and nutritional value per serving, as well as its percentage of the daily value (%DV), are displayed on the nutrition information panel. You can compare the product's energy and nutrient density to your daily requirements for calories and nutrients by using the nutrition facts panel. The following details on the nutrition facts panel are important to note:

- Serving size and servings per container: The number of servings that are present in a package is known as servings per container, while the serving size is the standardized amount of the product that is used to compute the nutrition facts.

You may measure and manage your portions to prevent overindulging by using the serving size and servings per container. You should divide or double the nutrition data based on how much you consume compared to the serving size. Additionally, you ought to make an effort to eat according to the suggested serving size or gauge your meals using your hand or visual signals.

- Calories: The number of calories indicates how much energy a single serving of the product contains. By burning more calories than you take in, the calories assist you control and restrict how many calories you eat. This is known as a negative energy balance. Products that are high in calories but poor in nutrients, such soda, chips, cookies, and candy, should be avoided or consumed in moderation. Instead, you should try to choose foods that are low in calories but high in nutrients, like fruits, vegetables, whole grains, lean proteins, and low-fat dairy.

- Nutrients: The nutrients indicate how much and what kind of macronutrients (proteins, fats, and carbs) and micronutrients (vitamins and minerals) are included in a single serving of the product, together with their percentage of the daily value (%DV). The percentage of a nutrient that a single serving of the product contains is indicated by the %DV in relation to the average adult's recommended daily intake. You can meet your daily nutrient needs and maintain a balance between macro and micronutrients with the aid of these nutrients. Aim for products low in sodium, sugar, trans fat, and saturated fat, which can lead to weight gain and other health issues, and high in fiber, protein, and complex carbs, which can increase your metabolism and help you feel fuller for longer. Additionally, you ought to select goods that are high in vitamins and minerals, like iron, zinc, magnesium, B12, C, D, and B12. These nutrients can assist a number of processes and functions related to weight loss.

- Examine the health claims: These are declarations, such as "low fat," "high fiber," or "lowers cholesterol," that highlight the connection between a nutrient or ingredient and a particular health issue or benefit. You can choose the health claims that best meet your demands and weight loss goals by using them to determine the product's possible advantages or disadvantages. You should be aware, though, that the product's overall quality or nutrition may not be reflected in the health claims, which are not necessarily true or trustworthy. As a result, you should compare goods and double-check the information by looking at the ingredients list and nutrition facts panel in addition to the health claims.

Chapter 4:
Effective Exercise Strategies
Cardiovascular Exercise

Exercise that promotes blood circulation and oxygen supply while raising heart rate and breathing is known as cardiovascular exercise, or cardio. Cardio improves your health and metabolism while burning fat and calories to help you lose weight. But in order to reap the greatest rewards from cardio, you must select the appropriate kind, level of intensity, frequency, and length of exercise, along with strength training and a well-balanced diet.

The kind of cardio you select will rely on your fitness level, goals, tastes, and the accessibility of facilities and equipment. Typical forms of cardio include:

- Running: This high-impact, high-intensity activity can help you lose a lot of weight and burn calories while also enhancing your bone density, endurance, and respiratory and cardiovascular systems. Running can be done on a track, trail, road, or indoor treadmill. To keep oneself interested and avoid boredom, you can change up the terrain, speed, and distance you travel.

- Cycling: Cycling is a low-impact, moderate-to-intense exercise that can increase muscle strength, endurance, and cardiovascular and respiratory health in addition to burning a moderate to high quantity of calories and fat. Cycling can be done on a bike, spin cycle, stationary bike, or outside in any weather. To keep yourself motivated and avoid getting bored, you can adjust the resistance, incline, and speed.

- Swimming: This low-impact, moderate-to-intense exercise can increase your endurance, muscular tone, and cardiovascular and respiratory health in addition to burning a moderate to high number of calories and fat. Swimming can be done in a lake, pool, or ocean utilizing a variety of strokes, including butterfly, backstroke, breaststroke, and freestyle. You can push yourself and avoid boredom by adjusting your speed, distance, and intensity.

- Rowing: This high-intensity, low-impact activity improves your cardiovascular and respiratory health, muscle power, endurance, and ability to burn a lot of calories and fat. You can row on an ergometer, on a rower, or on the water in a boat, kayak, or rowing machine. To keep yourself from getting bored, you can change the resistance, speed, and distance you go.

Your heart rate, or the number of times your heart beats per minute, determines the level of cardio you should do. You burn more fat and calories at a higher intensity when your heart rate is higher. On the other hand, you will need more recovery and a shorter length the more intense you are.

You can use your fingertips, a fitness tracker, or a heart rate monitor to determine your heart rate. The rate of perceived exertion (RPE) scale, which ranges from 1 (extremely easy) to 10 (very hard), can also be used to gauge how hard you feel you are working.

The frequency of your cardiac exercise is determined by your fitness level, goals, and schedule. It is generally advised to engage in moderate-intensity aerobic exercise for at least 150 minutes. 75 minutes per week of vigorous cardio exercise, or a mix of the two. Your weekly cardio can be split up into three or five sessions, based on your schedule and personal preferences. Additionally, you should give your body at least a day off in between workouts so that it can heal and adjust.

Your choice of cardio duration is influenced by your fitness level, goals, and intensity. You burn more fat and calories the longer you do it. On the other hand, you will require more stamina the longer you go without increasing your intensity. It is generally advised to perform cardiovascular exercise for at least 10 minutes per session, with the duration being gradually increased as fitness levels develop. Interval training, a technique that alternates between high- and low-intensity intervals, is another way to boost fat and calorie burning while enhancing performance and endurance.

Strength Training

Strength training, often known as resistance training, is a kind of exercise where you use weights, bands, or your own body weight as external resistance to work your muscles and build strength. By boosting your calorie expenditure, metabolism, and muscle mass while also enhancing your overall fitness and health, strength training can aid in weight loss. But in order to reap the full benefits of strength training, you must select the appropriate exercises, as well as the appropriate levels of intensity, frequency, and duration of training. Add to this a healthy diet and cardiovascular activity.

Your tastes, objectives, degree of fitness, and the accessibility of facilities and equipment all influence the strength training routines you select. Here are a few typical strength training exercises:

Exercises for the lower body that work your quadriceps, hamstrings, glutes, and core include squats. Weights like dumbbells, barbells, or kettlebells can be used for squat exercises or not. With your feet shoulder-width apart, drop your hips until your thighs are parallel to the floor, then push yourself back up to the starting position to do a squat. You can also carry the weight on your shoulders or in front of your chest.

- Lunges: A lower body workout, lunges develop your quadriceps, hamstrings, glutes, and core. Weights like dumbbells, barbells, or kettlebells can be used for lunge exercises or not. To execute a lunge, place your feet hip-width apart, support your weight on your shoulders or in front of your chest, and take a big step forward with one leg. Bend both knees until your back knee is almost touching the floor and your front thigh is parallel to the ground. Then, push yourself back up to the starting position and repeat with the other leg.

- Push-ups: A great upper body workout for your triceps, shoulders, core, and chest are push-ups. You can perform push-ups in a variety of ways, including diamond, incline, and decline. Put your hands on the floor slightly wider than your shoulders, extend your legs behind you, and maintain a straight torso from head to toe to complete a push-up. After bringing your chest nearly to the floor, raise it back up to the starting position.

- Pull-ups: A great upper body workout for your back, biceps, and forearms are pull-ups. You can perform pull-ups with or without a wide, narrow, or neutral grip. With your hands facing away from you and your arms fully stretched, grab a pull-up bar to complete a pull-up. After raising your chin above the bar, return to the beginning position by lowering yourself.

- Planks: A core workout that works your lower back, oblique, and abdominal muscles. Planks can be performed with or without side, reverse, or mountain climber variations. Lie on your forearms on the ground with your elbows beneath your shoulders to do a plank. Maintain a straight torso from head to toe and extend your legs behind you. Try not to sag or arch your back while you hold this position as long as you can.

The resistance, repetitions, and sets you employ for each exercise determine the strength training intensity you will select. Your body will burn more fat and calories at a higher intensity when the resistance, repetitions, and sets are increased. But the shorter the period and the greater the intensity, the more recovery you'll need. The rate of perceived exertion (RPE) scale, which is a subjective indicator of how hard you feel you are working, can be used to gauge the intensity of strength training. It ranges from 1 (very easy) to 10 (extremely hard).

Your schedule, fitness level, and goals will all influence how frequently your strength train. It is often advised to perform two or three strength training sessions on non-consecutive days each week. Depending on your schedule and tastes, you can split up your workouts into several muscle areas, such as upper body, lower body, or complete body.

Additionally, you should give yourself at least 48 hours of rest in between workouts so that your muscles can repair and strengthen.

The number and kind of exercises, as well as the intensity, frequency, and rest intervals used throughout each session, will determine how long you choose to do strength training. You burn more calories and fat for a longer period of time. But the longer it goes on, the less intense it is, and the more stamina you'll need. Strength training is generally advised to be done for at least 20 to 30 minutes each session, with the duration being gradually increased as fitness levels develop. Circuit training is another way to boost fat and calorie burning while enhancing performance and endurance. It involves switching between various activities with little to no downtime.

Flexibility and Mobility Exercises

Exercises that increase flexibility and mobility help your joints and muscles operate better and have a wider range of motion. activities for flexibility require stretching your muscles to lengthen and become more supple, and activities for mobility entail fully rotating your joints to enhance stability and lubrication. Exercises for flexibility and mobility can improve your posture, movement, and performance, help you avoid discomfort and injuries, and help you lose weight.

Because they make it easier and safer to conduct other forms of exercise, like strength training and cardio, flexibility and mobility activities are crucial for weight loss. By increasing your range of motion and flexibility, you can:

- Boost muscle recruitment and activation to help you gain more muscle mass and strength as well as burn more fat and calories.

- Become more balanced and aligned, which will help you keep good form and technique and lower your chance of falling or losing control.

Lowering your levels of muscle tension and stiffness can help you move more fluidly and pleasantly while preventing cramps or spasms.

- Strengthen your regeneration and recuperation, which might hasten your healing process and lessen discomfort and inflammation.

As an additional workout on your days off, or as a warm-up before your main workout, flexibility and mobility exercises can be performed. Additionally, you can include them in your regular regimen, for example, in the morning, at work, or right before bed. Exercises for increasing range of motion and flexibility can be done using a variety of equipment and techniques, including body weight, bands, straps, foam rollers, and massage balls.

Depending on your tastes and goals, you can also use several types of stretching, such as static, dynamic, or active stretching.

Exercises that improve mobility and flexibility include the following:

- Neck rolls are a mobility exercise that work the muscles in your upper back and neck. Sit or stand with your back straight and your shoulders relaxed to execute a neck roll. For ten to fifteen repetitions in each direction, slowly turn your head in a clockwise and counterclockwise circle.

One mobility exercise that works the muscles in your upper back and shoulders is the shoulder circle. With your arms out to your sides and your feet shoulder-width apart, you can perform shoulder circles. For ten to fifteen repetitions in each direction, slowly rotate your shoulders forward and backward while forming wide circles with your arms.

- Cat-cow stretch: This flexibility exercise strengthens your core and spine muscles. With your wrists under your shoulders and your knees under your hips, begin a cat-cow stretch on your hands and knees. Breathe in, arch your back, raise your tailbone and chest, and raise your gaze. This is the position of the cow. Take a breath out, turn your back, tuck your tailbone and chin in, and look down.

The cat position is this. Move with your breath as you switch between the two poses for ten to fifteen repetitions.

Stretching your hamstrings and lower back muscles is a great way to improve your flexibility. Sit on the floor with your back straight and your legs out in front of you to conduct a hamstring stretch. Without bending your knees, extend your arms forward and attempt, as best you can, to touch your toes. For two to three repetitions, hold the stretch for 15 to 30 seconds, then release it.

A flexibility exercise that works your hip flexor and quadriceps muscles is the hip flexor stretch. Stretch your hip flexors by kneeling on the floor with your left leg behind you and your right leg in front of you, both bent 90 degrees. Put your hands on your right leg and push your hips forward until your left thigh and hip start to stretch. After holding the stretch for 15 to 30 seconds, switch sides and do it twice or three times.

Chapter 5:
Combining Nutrition and Exercise for Weight Loss
Creating a Balanced Routine

A vital tactic to reaching your objectives and keeping your weight loss outcomes is developing a balanced routine. In addition to eating healthily and exercising frequently, a balanced routine includes managing your stress, sleep, and mental well-being. To help you create a healthy routine for weight loss, consider the following actions and advice:

- Set attainable and precise goals: Prior to embarking on your weight loss journey, you should decide on your objectives and the metrics you'll use to track your development. You should set SMART goals, which entails:

- Specific: Your objectives ought to be well-defined and specific. For example, "I want to run a 5K in 30 minutes" or "I want to lose 10 pounds in 3 months" are examples of goal-setting.

Measurable: Whether you use a scale, tape measure, fitness tracker, or journal, your goals should be measurable and observable.

- Achievable: Considering your present capabilities, resources, and constraints, your objectives have to be demanding yet reachable.

- Relevant: Your objectives should be in line with your values and motives, and they should hold personal significance for you.

- Time-bound: Your objectives ought to be accompanied with a deadline or time period, like "every week" or "by the end of the year."

- Plan your diet and exercise: After you've established your objectives, you need to schedule your meals and workouts according to your calorie and nutritional requirements, preferences, and availability. Your exercise and nutrition regimen should be:

- Balanced: Eat a range of foods from various dietary groups, such as fruits, vegetables, whole grains, lean meats, healthy fats, and low-fat dairy. Restrict or avoid foods rich in fat, sugar, salt, or calories, such as processed, fried, or fast food. Exercises that work your entire body and enhance your health and fitness should be a combination of aerobic, strength, and flexibility training.

- Moderate: To help you feel fuller for longer and avoid overeating, your diet should include adequate calories, but not too many, as well as foods high in fiber, protein, and complex carbs. You should choose an exercise regimen that is appropriate for your fitness level and goals, and that is tough but manageable.

- Consistent: Your workout and nutrition plan should be adhered to consistently, without interruption or change, and without being overly strict or constrictive. Along with keeping an eye on things, you should assess your outcomes and progress and modify your plan as necessary.

- Control your sleep and stress: In addition to following a healthy diet and exercising, you should also pay attention to your sleep and stress levels because they have an impact on your ability to lose weight and how you feel overall. The way you handle stress and sleep should be:

- Adequate: Sleep has a direct impact on your appetite, metabolism, energy, mood, and immune system. Aim for 7 to 9 hours of excellent sleep per night. As stress can lead to emotional eating, cravings, inflammation, poor sleep, and digestive issues, you should also make an effort to manage or lessen your stress.

Regular: Coffee, alcohol, nicotine, and screens should be avoided right before bed since these can interfere with both the quantity and quality of your sleep. Instead, you should attempt to keep a regular sleep and wake cycle. In order to reduce stress and soothe your body and mind, you could also try to practice relaxation techniques like breathing, yoga, meditation, massage, or engaging in fun activities like hobbies, music, or socializing.

- Supportive: Make sure your bedroom is cold, dark, and quiet. Keep distractions like light and noise to a minimum. Try to establish a pleasant and stress-relieving atmosphere.

If you struggle to fall asleep, manage your stress, or require assistance with your weight reduction journey, you should also make an effort to get support from your family, friends, or experts.

Setting Realistic Goals

A vital first step in achieving and maintaining your desired weight reduction outcomes is setting realistic goals. While realistic goals can increase your confidence, contentment, and adherence, unrealistic goals might cause you to feel frustrated, disappointed, and demotivated. Here are some pointers and actions to help you create reasonable weight loss goals:

Achievable, Measurable, Relevant, and Time-bound are the five SMART criteria that should be applied. You may more successfully outline your objectives and monitor your progress by using these criteria. For instance, you may state, "I want to lose 10 pounds in 3 months by following a balanced diet and exercising 3 times a week," as opposed to, "I want to lose weight."

- Start small and build up gradually: As your abilities and confidence grow, it's preferable to begin with modest, manageable objectives that you can accomplish fast and reliably. As you advance, you can progressively take on more challenging and demanding tasks. For instance, you may begin with walking for 30 minutes a day during your first month of training, and then progressively increase the distance, pace, and intensity. Rather than preparing for a marathon.

- Be adaptable and flexible: It's common to run across setbacks and barriers along your weight loss journey, such as injuries, plateaus, or life events. You can be flexible and adaptable to modify your goals and techniques in accordance with your present situation and needs, rather of giving up or feeling guilty. For instance, you may cut back on the frequency or intensity of your workouts if you have a hectic workweek; if you're injured, you could focus on your nutrition or move to a low-impact sport.

- appreciate your successes and treat yourself: No matter how big or small your accomplishments are, it's crucial to recognize and appreciate them. Treat yourself to something that brings you joy and helps you reach your weight reduction objectives. You may reward yourself with a massage, a new wardrobe, or a movie night, for instance. You could also use social media to tell your loved ones about your accomplishments. This can support your good actions and help you keep your motivation and excitement levels high.

- Seek support and feedback: Getting support and input from people who can motivate, inspire, and hold you responsible for your objectives is beneficial. You can look for a weight loss companion, a coach, or a mentor. You can also enroll in a fitness class, an online community, or a weight loss organization.

A personal trainer, nutritionist, or healthcare practitioner are additional resources you might consult for assistance and direction.

Tracking Progress and Adjustments

Any weight loss journey must include tracking progress and alterations since it allows you to keep an eye on your outcomes, assess your methods, and adjust as necessary. Monitoring your development and making any corrections can also help you stay accountable, motivated, and goal-focused. Observing progress and making necessary modifications to lose weight can be done in the following ways:

- Select your metrics and techniques: Prior to embarking on your weight loss journey, you must determine the metrics and techniques you will use to monitor your development and make necessary adjustments. Typical measurements and techniques include:

- Weight: Since it indicates how much you have gained or lost over time, weight is the most obvious and straightforward indicator to track your weight loss. You can weigh yourself using a scale, ideally first thing in the morning, when you're not eating or drinking, and when you're not wearing a lot of clothes. Additionally, since your weight can vary every day owing to a variety of causes like water retention, hormone fluctuations, or muscle building, you should track your weight in a notebook, calendar, or app and determine your weekly or monthly average.

- Body fat percentage: This measure indicates how much of your weight is made up of lean mass and fat, making it a more precise and thorough way to monitor your weight loss. Your body fat % can be calculated using a variety of tools, including internet calculators, calipers, DEXA scans, and bioelectrical impedance scales. Additionally, you should track your body fat % using a notebook, calendar, or app. Then, you should compare it to other metrics and your weight. While your weight may not vary significantly, a decrease in your body fat percentage could mean that you are growing muscle and losing fat.

- Body measurements: Since they reflect changes in your body's size and shape, body measurements are another helpful tool to monitor your weight loss. Measure your arms, thighs, hips, chest, and waist with a tape measure, then record the measurements in a diary, calendar, or app. A weight loss chart is another useful tool for monitoring your progress. It allows you to compare your measurements with your weight and body fat percentage. If your measures drop, it may be an indication that you are getting more toned and dropping inches.

- Photos: Since they display how your appearance and confidence are growing, photos are a motivating and visual way to monitor your weight loss. Every week or month, you can snap pictures of yourself in the same outfit, perspective, lighting, and stance and save them in an app, calendar, or notebook. Your images may show changes that you might not see otherwise, such better posture, less cellulite, or enhanced facial characteristics. You can use a weight loss chart to track your progress and compare your photos with your other metrics.

- Evaluate your progress and modifications: Depending on your goals and preferences, you should assess your progress and adjustments on a regular basis, ideally once a week or once a month, after you have selected your metrics and methods. You can examine your statistics and trends using a notebook, calendar, or app to see whether you are on track with your objectives or whether any adjustments need to be made. A weight loss chart is another useful tool for tracking your progress and making adjustments. It also shows you how your approaches and metrics relate to one another and to your overall weight reduction. Based on your age, gender, height, weight, exercise level, and weight loss objective, you may also use a weight loss calculator to determine your calorie and nutrient needs, as well as your ideal weight and body fat percentage.

- Make adjustments as necessary: To maximize your weight loss outcomes and get beyond any obstacles or plateaus, you can make necessary alterations to your food, exercise routine, and way of life based on your evaluation of your progress and modifications. Typical alterations include:

Diet: To fit your current needs and tastes, you can modify your calorie intake, macronutrient ratio, portion size, meal frequency, and timing. To determine which diet is best for you, you can also experiment with a variety of approaches, including Mediterranean, low-carb, high-protein, and intermittent fasting. To track your food and nutrient intake and see how it affects your weight reduction, you can also use a food diary, tracker, or app.

- Exercise: You can modify the type, intensity, frequency, and duration of your workouts to meet your goals and present level of fitness. Exercises including aerobic, strength, flexibility, and high-intensity interval training (HIIT) can all be tried to find which suits you best. Additionally, you can track your workout performance and calorie expenditure with a fitness tracker, watch, or app to observe how they impact your weight reduction.

- Lifestyle: You can modify your sleep, stress level, and mental state to better fit your needs and overall wellbeing. To find what works best for you, you can also experiment with various lifestyle modifications, such as yoga, meditation, massages, or new hobbies. Additionally, you can track the quantity and quality of your sleep with a watch, app, or sleep tracker to observe how it affects your weight loss.

Chapter 6:

Some Healthy Recipes for Weight Loss

Breakfast recipes

1. Spinach & Egg Scramble with Raspberries

Ingredients:

- 2 teaspoons canola oil

- 2 cups baby spinach

- 4 large eggs, lightly beaten

- 1/4 teaspoon salt

- 1/4 teaspoon black pepper

- 2 slices whole-wheat bread, toasted

- 1 cup fresh raspberries

Preparation:

- Heat oil in a large nonstick skillet over medium-high heat. Add spinach and cook, stirring, until wilted, about 2 minutes.

- Add eggs, salt, and pepper and cook, stirring, until set about 4 minutes.

- Divide the egg mixture and toast among two plates. Top with raspberries and serve.

Nutritional value (per serving):

- Calories: 297

- Fat: 16 g

- Carbohydrates: 25 g

- Fiber: 8 g

- Protein: 18 g

Cooking time: 10 minutes

2. Berry-Almond Smoothie Bowl

Ingredients:

- 3/4 cup frozen blueberries

- 3/4 cup frozen raspberries

- 1/4 cup unsweetened almond milk

- 2 tablespoons almond butter

- 1 tablespoon chia seeds

- 1/4 teaspoon vanilla extract

- 1/4 teaspoon ground cinnamon

- Toppings: sliced almonds, fresh berries, shredded coconut, granola, etc.

Preparation:

- Combine blueberries, raspberries, almond milk, almond butter, chia seeds, vanilla, and cinnamon in a blender and blend until smooth and thick, scraping down the sides as needed.

- Transfer to a bowl and sprinkle with your desired toppings. Enjoy with a spoon.

Nutritional value (per serving):

- Calories: 386

- Fat: 23 g

- Carbohydrates: 40 g

- Fiber: 15 g

- Protein: 11 g

Cooking time: 5 minutes

3. Sriracha, Egg & Avocado Overnight Oats

Ingredients:

- 1/2 cup old-fashioned rolled oats

- 1/2 cup water

- 1/4 teaspoon salt

- 1/4 teaspoon black pepper

- 1/4 teaspoon garlic powder

- 1/4 teaspoon onion powder

- 1 teaspoon sriracha sauce, plus more for serving

- 1 large egg

- 1/4 avocado, sliced

- 2 tablespoons chopped fresh cilantro

Preparation:

- Combine oats, water, salt, pepper, garlic powder, onion powder, and sriracha in a small microwave-safe bowl. Cover and refrigerate overnight.

- In the morning, microwave the oat mixture on high until hot and thickened, about 2 minutes, stirring once halfway.

- In a small nonstick skillet over medium-high heat, spray some cooking spray and crack the egg. Cook until the white is set and the yolk is runny, about 3 minutes, or flip and cook longer for a firmer yolk.

- Top the oat mixture with the egg, avocado, cilantro, and more sriracha if desired. Enjoy with a fork.

Nutritional value (per serving):

- Calories: 337

- Fat: 16 g

- Carbohydrates: 39 g

- Fiber: 9 g

- Protein: 14 g

Cooking time: 10 minutes

4. Peanut Energy Bars

Ingredients:

- 1/4 cup unsalted dry-roasted peanuts

- 1/4 cup roasted sunflower seeds

- 2 tablespoons sesame seeds

- 2 tablespoons flaxseeds

- 1 cup raisins

- 1/2 cup pitted dates

- 1/4 cup peanut butter

- 1/4 cup honey

- 1/4 teaspoon salt

- Cooking spray

Preparation:

- Preheat oven to 325°F. Line an 8-inch-square baking pan with parchment paper and coat with cooking spray.

- In a food processor, pulse peanuts, sunflower seeds, sesame seeds, and flaxseeds until coarsely chopped. Transfer to a large bowl and stir in raisins and dates.

- In a small saucepan over low heat, combine peanut butter, honey, and salt and cook, stirring, until smooth and bubbly, about 2 minutes.

- Pour the peanut butter mixture over the fruit and nut mixture and stir well to combine. Press the mixture evenly into the prepared pan and bake until lightly browned about 25 minutes.

- Let the bars cool completely in the pan on a wire rack before cutting into 16 pieces. Store in an airtight container at room temperature for up to 5 days, or freeze for up to 3 months.

Nutritional value (per serving):

- Calories: 149

- Fat: 7 g

- Carbohydrates: 21 g

- Fiber: 3 g

- Protein: 4 g

Cooking time: 35 minutes

5. Avocado & Kale Omelet

Ingredients:

- 2 teaspoons extra-virgin olive oil

- 2 cups chopped kale

- 1/4 teaspoon salt, divided

- 4 large eggs

- 2 tablespoons water

- 1/4 teaspoon black pepper

- 1/4 cup shredded cheddar cheese

- 1/4 avocado, diced

Preparation:

- Heat oil in a large nonstick skillet over medium-high heat. Add kale and 1/8 teaspoon salt and cook, stirring, until wilted, about 4 minutes. Transfer to a plate and keep warm.

- In a small bowl, whisk eggs, water, pepper, and the remaining 1/8 teaspoon salt. Coat the same skillet with cooking spray and heat over medium heat. Pour the egg mixture into the skillet and cook, lifting the edges with a spatula to let the uncooked egg flow underneath, until almost set, about 3 minutes.

- Sprinkle cheese over half of the omelet and fold the other half over the cheese. Cook until the cheese is melted, about 1 minute more. Cut into two pieces and serve with the kale and avocado.

Nutritional value (per serving):

- Calories: 286

- Fat: 21 g

- Carbohydrates: 9 g

- Fiber: 3 g

- Protein: 18 g

Cooking time: 15 minutes

6. Greek Yogurt Parfait with Granola and Berries

Ingredients:

- 1 cup plain low-fat Greek yogurt

- 1/4 cup low-fat granola

- 1/2 cup fresh or frozen mixed berries

- 1 tablespoon honey or maple syrup (optional)

Preparation:

- In a small bowl or glass, layer half of the yogurt, granola, and berries. Repeat with the remaining yogurt, granola, and berries.

- Drizzle with honey or maple syrup if desired. Enjoy with a spoon.

Nutritional value (per serving):

- Calories: 310

- Fat: 6 g

- Carbohydrates: 47 g

- Fiber: 6 g

- Protein: 20 g

Cooking time: 5 minutes

7. Banana-Nut Waffles

Ingredients:

- 1 1/4 cups whole-wheat flour

- 2 teaspoons baking powder

- 1/4 teaspoon salt

- 1/4 teaspoon cinnamon

- 1 cup low-fat milk

- 2 large eggs

- 2 tablespoons canola oil

- 2 tablespoons brown sugar

- 1 ripe banana, mashed

- 1/4 cup chopped walnuts

- Cooking spray

- Toppings: sliced banana, maple syrup, peanut butter, etc.

Preparation:

- Preheat a waffle iron and coat with cooking spray.

- In a large bowl, whisk together the flour, baking powder, salt, and cinnamon.

- In a medium bowl, whisk together the milk, eggs, oil, and brown sugar. Stir in the mashed banana and walnuts.

- Add the wet ingredients to the dry ingredients and stir until just combined. Do not overmix.

- Spoon about 1/4 cup of the batter onto the waffle iron and cook until golden and crisp, about 3 to 4 minutes. Repeat with the remaining batter.

- Serve the waffles with your desired toppings.

Nutritional value (per serving):

- Calories: 278

- Fat: 13 g

- Carbohydrates: 35 g

- Fiber: 4 g

- Protein: 9 g

Cooking time: 20 minutes

8. Spinach & Cheese Breakfast Sandwich

Ingredients:

- 1 teaspoon olive oil

- 2 cups baby spinach

- 1/4 teaspoon garlic powder

- Salt and pepper to taste

- 1 large egg

- 1 slice of reduced-fat cheddar cheese

- 1 whole-wheat English muffin, split and toasted

Preparation:

- Heat oil in a small nonstick skillet over medium-high heat. Add spinach and garlic powder and cook, stirring, until wilted, about 2 minutes. Season with salt and pepper and transfer to a plate.

- In the same skillet, spray some cooking spray and crack the egg. Cook until the white is set and the yolk is runny, about 3 minutes, or flip and cook longer for a firmer yolk.

- Place the cheese on the bottom half of the English muffin and top with the egg and spinach. Cover with the top half of the muffin and enjoy.

Nutritional value (per serving):

- Calories: 265

- Fat: 12 g

- Carbohydrates: 27 g

- Fiber: 4 g

- Protein: 16 g

Cooking time: 10 minutes

9. Apple-Cinnamon Overnight Oats

Ingredients:

- 1/2 cup old-fashioned rolled oats

- 1/2 cup unsweetened almond milk

- 1/4 cup plain low-fat Greek yogurt

- 1/4 teaspoon vanilla extract

- 1/4 teaspoon ground cinnamon

- 1/8 teaspoon ground nutmeg

- 1 small apple, chopped

- 1 tablespoon chopped pecans

- 1 teaspoon honey or maple syrup (optional)

Preparation:

- In a small bowl or jar, stir together the oats, almond milk, yogurt, vanilla, cinnamon, and nutmeg. Cover and refrigerate overnight.

- In the morning, stir in the apple, pecans, and honey or maple syrup if desired. Enjoy cold or warm in the microwave.

Nutritional value (per serving):

- Calories: 295

- Fat: 9 g

- Carbohydrates: 46 g

- Fiber: 8 g

- Protein: 12 g

Cooking time: 5 minutes

10. Veggie & Hummus Breakfast Wrap

Ingredients:

- 1 whole-wheat tortilla (8-inch)

- 2 tablespoons hummus

- 1/4 cup shredded carrots

- 1/4 cup sliced cucumber

- 1/4 cup sliced red bell pepper

- 2 tablespoons crumbled feta cheese

- 1 tablespoon chopped fresh parsley

Preparation:

- Spread the hummus evenly over the tortilla. Top with the carrots, cucumber, bell pepper, feta and parsley.

- Roll up the tortilla and cut it in half. Enjoy with a glass of water or low-fat milk.

Nutritional value (per serving):

- Calories: 258

- Fat: 10 g

- Carbohydrates: 35 g

- Fiber: 7 g

- Protein: 10 g

Cooking time: 10 minutes

Lunch recipes for weight loss

1. Chicken and Vegetable Stir-Fry

Ingredients:

- 1 tablespoon cornstarch

- 1/4 cup low sodium soy sauce

- 1/4 cup water

- 1 tablespoon honey

- 1 teaspoon sesame oil

- 1/4 teaspoon red pepper flakes

- 1 tablespoon canola oil

- 1 pound boneless, skinless chicken breasts, cut into thin strips

- 2 cups broccoli florets

- 1 cup sliced carrots

- 1/4 cup sliced green onions

Preparation:

- In a small bowl, whisk together the cornstarch, soy sauce, water, honey, sesame oil, and red pepper flakes until smooth. Set aside.

- Heat the canola oil in a large skillet over high heat. Add the chicken and cook, stirring, until browned and cooked through, about 10 minutes. Transfer to a plate and keep warm.

- In the same skillet, add the broccoli, carrots, and green onions and cook, stirring, until crisp-tender, about 5 minutes.

- Stir in the sauce and bring to a boil. Cook, stirring, until thickened, about 2 minutes.

- Return the chicken to the skillet and toss to coat with the sauce. Serve hot with brown rice or quinoa if desired.

Nutritional value (per serving):

- Calories: 264

- Fat: 8 g

- Carbohydrates: 18 g

- Fiber: 3 g

- Protein: 31 g

Cooking time: 25 minutes

2. Mediterranean Salad with Tuna

Ingredients:

- 4 cups mixed salad greens

- 1/4 cup chopped fresh parsley

- 2 tablespoons chopped fresh mint

- 2 tablespoons lemon juice

- 2 tablespoons olive oil

- Salt and pepper to taste

- 1 (5-ounce) can tuna in water, drained and flaked

- 1/4 cup sliced black olives

- 1/4 cup crumbled feta cheese

- 2 whole-wheat pita bread, cut into wedges

Preparation:

- In a large bowl, toss the salad greens, parsley, mint, lemon juice, olive oil, salt and pepper until well combined.

- Divide the salad among four plates and top with tuna, olives, and feta cheese.

- Serve with pita bread wedges.

Nutritional value (per serving):

- Calories: 287

- Fat: 15 g

- Carbohydrates: 23 g

- Fiber: 4 g

- Protein: 18 g

Cooking time: 15 minutes

3. Turkey and Bean Chili

Ingredients:

- 1 tablespoon canola oil

- 1 onion, chopped

- 2 cloves garlic, minced

- 1 pound lean ground turkey

- 2 tablespoons chili powder

- 1 teaspoon cumin

- 1/4 teaspoon salt

- 1/4 teaspoon black pepper

- 1 (15-ounce) can tomato sauce

- 1 (14.5-ounce) can diced tomatoes

- 1 (15-ounce) can black beans, rinsed and drained

- 1/4 cup chopped fresh cilantro

Preparation:

- Heat the oil in a large pot over medium-high heat. Add the onion and garlic and cook, stirring, until soft, about 5 minutes.

- Add the turkey and cook, breaking it up with a wooden spoon, until browned and cooked through, about 10 minutes.

- Stir in the chili powder, cumin, salt, pepper, tomato sauce, diced tomatoes and black beans. Bring to a boil, then reduce the heat and simmer, uncovered, until slightly thickened, about 15 minutes.

- Stir in the cilantro and serve with shredded cheese, sour cream, or avocado if desired.

Nutritional value (per serving):

- Calories: 292

- Fat: 9 g

- Carbohydrates: 28 g

- Fiber: 9 g

- Protein: 28 g

Cooking time: 35 minutes

4. Roasted Vegetable and Hummus Sandwich

Ingredients:

- 1 small zucchini, sliced

- 1 small yellow squash, sliced

- 1 small red onion, sliced

- 1 red bell pepper, sliced

- 2 tablespoons olive oil

- Salt and pepper to taste

- 4 whole-wheat sandwich rolls, split and toasted

- 1/4 cup hummus

- 4 lettuce leaves

- 4 slices tomato

Preparation:

- Preheat oven to 425°F. Line a baking sheet with parchment paper.

- In a large bowl, toss the zucchini, squash, onion, and bell pepper with the olive oil, salt, and pepper. Spread in a single layer on the prepared baking sheet. Roast for 20 minutes, turning once, until tender and browned.

- Spread the hummus evenly over the bottom halves of the rolls. Top with the roasted vegetables, lettuce, and tomato. Cover with the top halves of the rolls and cut in half. Serve warm or at room temperature.

Nutritional value (per serving):

- Calories: 281

- Fat: 11 g

- Carbohydrates: 40 g

- Fiber: 8 g

- Protein: 10 g

Cooking time: 30 minutes

5. Greek Chicken and Quinoa Salad

Ingredients:

- 1/4 cup lemon juice

- 2 tablespoons olive oil

- 2 teaspoons dried oregano

- 1/4 teaspoon salt

- 1/4 teaspoon black pepper

- 1 pound boneless, skinless chicken breasts, cut into bite-sized pieces

- 2 cups cooked quinoa

- 2 cups chopped cucumber

- 1 cup halved cherry tomatoes

- 1/4 cup sliced black olives

- 1/4 cup crumbled feta cheese

- 2 tablespoons chopped fresh parsley

Preparation:

- In a small bowl, whisk together the lemon juice, olive oil, oregano, salt and pepper. Reserve 2 tablespoons of the dressing and set aside.

- In a large zip-top bag, add the chicken and the remaining dressing and seal. Refrigerate for at least 30 minutes or up to 4 hours.

- Preheat a grill or broiler to high. Remove the chicken from the marinade and discard the marinade. Grill or broil the chicken, turning once, until cooked through about 10 minutes.

- In a large bowl, toss the quinoa, cucumber, tomatoes, olives, feta, and parsley with the reserved dressing. Serve with the chicken.

Nutritional value (per serving):

- Calories: 361

- Fat: 15 g

- Carbohydrates: 28 g

- Fiber: 4 g

- Protein: 32 g

Cooking time: 45 minutes

6. Roasted Vegetable and Quinoa Salad

Ingredients:

- 2 cups cherry tomatoes, halved

- 2 cups cauliflower florets

- 2 cups Brussels sprouts, trimmed and halved

- 2 tablespoons olive oil

- Salt and pepper to taste

- 2 cups cooked quinoa

- 1/4 cup chopped fresh parsley

- 2 tablespoons lemon juice

- 2 teaspoons Dijon mustard

- 1/4 teaspoon garlic powder

Preparation:

- Preheat oven to 425°F. Line a baking sheet with parchment paper.

- In a large bowl, toss the tomatoes, cauliflower, and Brussels sprouts with the olive oil, salt, and pepper. Spread in a single layer on the prepared baking sheet. Roast for 25 minutes, stirring once, until tender and browned.

- In a small bowl, whisk together the parsley, lemon juice, mustard, and garlic powder. Season with salt and pepper to taste.

- In a large serving bowl, toss the quinoa with the roasted vegetables and the dressing. Serve warm or cold.

Nutritional value (per serving):

- Calories: 279

- Fat: 11 g

- Carbohydrates: 40 g

- Fiber: 9 g

- Protein: 10 g

Cooking time: 35 minutes

7. Turkey and Avocado Sandwich

Ingredients:

- 4 slices whole-wheat bread, toasted

- 2 tablespoons mayonnaise

- 4 ounces sliced turkey breast

- 4 lettuce leaves

- 1/4 avocado, sliced

- 1/4 teaspoon salt

- 1/4 teaspoon black pepper

Preparation:

- Spread the mayonnaise evenly over two slices of bread. Top with the turkey, lettuce, and avocado. Season with salt and pepper. Cover with the remaining slices of bread and cut in half. Serve with baby carrots or apple slices if desired.

Nutritional value (per serving):

- Calories: 287

- Fat: 13 g

- Carbohydrates: 29 g

- Fiber: 6 g

- Protein: 18 g

Cooking time: 10 minutes

8. Asian Chicken and Cabbage Salad

Ingredients:

- 1/4 cup rice vinegar

- 2 tablespoons soy sauce

- 1 tablespoon honey

- 1 tablespoon sesame oil

- 1 teaspoon grated ginger

- 1/4 teaspoon red pepper flakes

- 3 cups shredded cooked chicken

- 4 cups shredded green cabbage

- 2 cups shredded red cabbage

- 1/4 cup chopped fresh cilantro

- 2 tablespoons toasted sesame seeds

Preparation:

- In a small bowl, whisk together the vinegar, soy sauce, honey, sesame oil, ginger and red pepper flakes. Set aside.

- In a large bowl, toss the chicken, green cabbage, red cabbage, and cilantro. Drizzle with the dressing and toss to coat. Sprinkle with the sesame seeds and serve.

Nutritional value (per serving):

- Calories: 263

- Fat: 10 g

- Carbohydrates: 18 g

- Fiber: 4 g

- Protein: 27 g

Cooking time: 15 minutes

9. Tomato and White Bean Soup

Ingredients:

- 2 teaspoons olive oil

- 1 onion, chopped

- 2 cloves garlic, minced

- 4 cups low sodium vegetable broth

- 2 (14.5-ounce) cans of diced tomatoes

- 1 (15-ounce) can of white beans, rinsed and drained

- 2 teaspoons dried basil

- 1/4 teaspoon salt

- 1/4 teaspoon black pepper

- 2 cups baby spinach

Preparation:

- Heat the oil in a large pot over medium-high heat. Add the onion and garlic and cook, stirring, until soft, about 5 minutes.

- Add the broth, tomatoes, beans, basil, salt and pepper, and bring to a boil. Reduce the heat and simmer, uncovered, until slightly thickened, about 15 minutes.

- Stir in the spinach and cook until wilted about 2 minutes. Serve with whole-wheat bread or crackers if desired.

Nutritional value (per serving):

- Calories: 181

- Fat: 3 g

- Carbohydrates: 31 g

- Fiber: 9 g

- Protein: 10 g

Cooking time: 25 minutes

10. Greek Chicken and Orzo Salad

Ingredients:

- 1/4 cup lemon juice

- 2 tablespoons olive oil

- 2 teaspoons dried oregano

- 1/4 teaspoon salt

- 1/4 teaspoon black pepper

- 1 pound boneless, skinless chicken breasts, cut into bite-sized pieces

- 2 cups cooked orzo

- 2 cups chopped cucumber

- 1 cup halved cherry tomatoes

- 1/4 cup sliced black olives

- 1/4 cup crumbled feta cheese

- 2 tablespoons chopped fresh parsley

Preparation:

- In a small bowl, whisk together the lemon juice, olive oil, oregano, salt and pepper. Reserve 2 tablespoons of the dressing and set aside.

- In a large zip-top bag, add the chicken and the remaining dressing and seal. Refrigerate for at least 30 minutes or up to 4 hours.

- Preheat a grill or broiler to high. Remove the chicken from the marinade and discard the marinade. Grill or broil the chicken, turning once, until cooked through about 10 minutes.

- In a large bowl, toss the orzo, cucumber, tomatoes, olives, feta, and parsley with the reserved dressing. Serve with the chicken.

Nutritional value (per serving):

- Calories: 361

- Fat: 15 g

- Carbohydrates: 28 g

- Fiber: 4 g

- Protein: 32 g

Cooking time: 45 minutes

1. Salmon and Roasted Vegetable Salad

Ingredients:

- 4 (4-ounce) salmon fillets

- 2 tablespoons lemon juice

- Salt and pepper to taste

- 4 cups baby spinach

- 2 cups cherry tomatoes, halved

- 2 cups cauliflower florets

- 2 tablespoons olive oil

- 1/4 cup plain low-fat Greek yogurt

- 2 tablespoons chopped fresh dill

- 1 teaspoon Dijon mustard

Preparation:

- Preheat oven to 425°F. Line a baking sheet with parchment paper.

- Place the salmon on the prepared baking sheet and drizzle with 1 tablespoon of lemon juice. Season with salt and pepper. Bake for 15 minutes or until the fish flakes easily with a fork.

- In a large bowl, toss the spinach, tomatoes, and cauliflower with the olive oil, salt, and pepper. Spread in a single layer on another baking sheet and roast for 20 minutes, stirring once, until tender and browned.

- In a small bowl, whisk together the yogurt, dill, mustard, and the remaining 1 tablespoon of lemon juice. Season with salt and pepper to taste.

- Divide the salad among four plates and top with the salmon. Drizzle with the yogurt dressing and serve.

Nutritional value (per serving):

- Calories: 328

- Fat: 18 g

- Carbohydrates: 14 g

- Fiber: 4 g

- Protein: 31 g

Cooking time: 35 minutes

2. Spaghetti Squash and Meatballs

Ingredients:

- 1 medium spaghetti squash (about 3 pounds)

- 1 pound lean ground turkey

- 1/4 cup grated Parmesan cheese

- 2 tablespoons chopped fresh parsley

- 1 teaspoon garlic powder

- Salt and pepper to taste

- 2 cups marinara sauce

- 1/4 cup shredded mozzarella cheese

Preparation:

- Preheat oven to 375°F. Cut the spaghetti squash in half and scoop out the seeds. Place the squash halves cut-side down on a baking sheet and bake for 45 minutes or until tender.

- In a large bowl, combine the turkey, Parmesan, parsley, garlic powder, salt and pepper. Shape into 16 meatballs and place on another baking sheet. Bake for 20 minutes or until cooked through.

- In a small saucepan over medium heat, warm the marinara sauce until bubbly.

- Using a fork, scrape the spaghetti squash strands into a large bowl. Divide among four plates and top with the meatballs and sauce. Sprinkle with mozzarella cheese and serve.

Nutritional value (per serving):

- Calories: 365

- Fat: 15 g

- Carbohydrates: 32 g

- Fiber: 7 g

- Protein: 31 g

Cooking time: 65 minutes

3. Chicken and Vegetable Curry

Ingredients:

- 1 tablespoon canola oil

- 1 onion, chopped

- 2 cloves garlic, minced

- 1 tablespoon curry powder

- 1 teaspoon cumin

- 1/4 teaspoon salt

- 1/4 teaspoon black pepper

- 1 (14-ounce) can light coconut milk

- 1 (14.5-ounce) can diced tomatoes

- 1 pound boneless, skinless chicken breasts, cut into bite-sized pieces

- 2 cups green beans, trimmed and cut into 1-inch pieces

- 2 cups cooked brown rice

Preparation:

- Heat the oil in a large skillet over medium-high heat. Add the onion and garlic and cook, stirring, until soft, about 5 minutes.

- Stir in the curry powder, cumin, salt and pepper and cook, stirring, for 1 minute.

- Add the coconut milk and tomatoes and bring to a boil. Reduce the heat and simmer, uncovered, for 10 minutes, stirring occasionally.

- Add the chicken and green beans and simmer, covered, until the chicken is cooked through and the green beans are tender, about 15 minutes.

- Serve the curry over the rice.

Nutritional value (per serving):

- Calories: 386

- Fat: 13 g

- Carbohydrates: 42 g

- Fiber: 7 g

- Protein: 29 g

Cooking time: 40 minutes

4. Vegetable and Bean Quesadillas

Ingredients:

- 1 tablespoon olive oil

- 1 red bell pepper, chopped

- 1 zucchini, chopped

- 1/4 teaspoon salt

- 1/4 teaspoon black pepper

- 1 (15-ounce) can black beans, rinsed and drained

- 1/4 cup salsa

- 8 (6-inch) whole-wheat tortillas

- 1 cup shredded cheddar cheese

- Cooking spray

Preparation:

- Heat the oil in a large skillet over medium-high heat. Add the bell pepper, zucchini, salt, and pepper and cook, stirring, until crisp-tender, about 10 minutes.

- In a small saucepan over low heat, mash the beans with a fork and stir in the salsa. Cook, stirring, until warm, about 5 minutes.

- Preheat a grill or broiler to high. Spread the bean mixture evenly over four tortillas and sprinkle with cheese. Top with the remaining tortillas and press lightly to seal.

- Coat both sides of the quesadillas with cooking spray and grill or broil, turning once, until golden and crisp, about 5 minutes.

- Cut into wedges and serve with sour cream, guacamole, or more salsa if desired.

Nutritional value (per serving):

- Calories: 366

- Fat: 14 g

- Carbohydrates: 48 g

- Fiber: 12 g

- Protein: 18 g

Cooking time: 25 minutes

5. Beef and Broccoli Stir-Fry

Ingredients:

- 1/4 cup low sodium soy sauce

- 2 tablespoons cornstarch

- 1 tablespoon honey

- 1 teaspoon sesame oil

- 1/4 teaspoon red pepper flakes

- 1 pound sirloin steak, thinly sliced

- 2 teaspoons canola oil

- 4 cups broccoli florets

- 2 cloves garlic, minced

- 2 teaspoons grated ginger

- 2 cups cooked brown rice

Preparation:

- In a small bowl, whisk together the soy sauce, cornstarch, honey, sesame oil, and red pepper flakes until smooth. Set aside.

- In a large zip-top bag, add the steak and 2 tablespoons of the sauce and seal. Refrigerate for at least 30 minutes or up to 4 hours.

- Heat the canola oil in a large nonstick skillet over high heat. Remove the steak from the marinade and discard the marinade. Cook, stirring, until browned and cooked to your liking, about 10 minutes. Transfer to a plate and keep warm.

- In the same skillet, add the broccoli, garlic, ginger, and 1/4 cup water and cook, stirring, until crisp-tender, about 5 minutes.

- Stir in the remaining sauce and bring to a boil. Cook, stirring, until thickened, about 2 minutes.

- Return the steak to the skillet and toss to coat with the sauce. Serve over the rice.

Nutritional value (per serving):

- Calories: 387

- Fat: 11 g

- Carbohydrates: 44 g

- Fiber: 5 g

- Protein: 31 g

Cooking time: 45 minutes

6. Spicy Shrimp and Vegetable Stir-Fry

Ingredients:

- 1/4 cup low sodium soy sauce

- 2 tablespoons rice vinegar

- 1 tablespoon honey

- 1 tablespoon cornstarch

- 1/4 teaspoon red pepper flakes

- 1 pound large shrimp, peeled and deveined

- 2 teaspoons canola oil

- 2 cups snow peas

- 1 cup sliced mushrooms

- 2 cloves garlic, minced

- 2 teaspoons grated ginger

- 2 cups cooked brown rice

Preparation:

- In a small bowl, whisk together the soy sauce, vinegar, honey, cornstarch, and red pepper flakes until smooth. Set aside.

- In a large zip-top bag, add the shrimp and 2 tablespoons of the sauce and seal. Refrigerate for at least 15 minutes or up to 1 hour.

- Heat the oil in a large nonstick skillet over high heat. Remove the shrimp from the marinade and discard the marinade. Cook, stirring, until pink and cooked through, about 5 minutes. Transfer to a plate and keep warm.

- In the same skillet, add the snow peas, mushrooms, garlic, ginger, and 1/4 cup water and cook, stirring, until crisp-tender, about 10 minutes.

- Stir in the remaining sauce and bring to a boil. Cook, stirring, until thickened, about 2 minutes.

- Return the shrimp to the skillet and toss to coat with the sauce. Serve over the rice.

Nutritional value (per serving):

- Calories: 339

- Fat: 6 g

- Carbohydrates: 46 g

- Fiber: 4 g

- Protein: 28 g

Cooking time: 35 minutes

7. Roasted Chicken and Vegetable Sheet-Pan Dinner

Ingredients:

- 4 (4-ounce) boneless, skinless chicken breasts

- 2 tablespoons olive oil

- 2 teaspoons dried rosemary

- Salt and pepper to taste

- 4 cups baby potatoes, halved

- 4 cups Brussels sprouts, trimmed and halved

- 2 cups baby carrots

- 1/4 cup balsamic vinegar

- 2 tablespoons honey

Preparation:

- Preheat oven to 425°F. Line a baking sheet with parchment paper.

- Rub the chicken with 1 tablespoon of olive oil, 1 teaspoon of rosemary, salt and pepper. Place on the prepared baking sheet and bake for 15 minutes.

- In a large bowl, toss the potatoes, Brussels sprouts, and carrots with the remaining olive oil, rosemary, salt, and pepper. Add to the baking sheet with the chicken and bake for another 15 minutes or until the chicken is cooked through and the vegetables are tender.

- In a small saucepan over medium-high heat, whisk together the vinegar and honey and bring to a boil. Reduce the heat and simmer, stirring, until slightly thickened, about 10 minutes.

- Drizzle the balsamic glaze over the chicken and vegetables and serve.

Nutritional value (per serving):

- Calories: 387

- Fat: 10 g

- Carbohydrates: 51 g

- Fiber: 8 g

- Protein: 30 g

Cooking time: 40 minutes

8. Vegetable and Cheese Frittata

Ingredients:

- 8 large eggs

- 1/4 cup low-fat milk

- Salt and pepper to taste

- 2 teaspoons olive oil

- 1 onion, chopped

- 2 cups chopped spinach

- 1 cup cherry tomatoes, halved

- 1/4 cup shredded cheddar cheese

Preparation:

- Preheat oven to 375°F. In a medium bowl, whisk together the eggs, milk, salt and pepper. Set aside.

- Heat the oil in a 10-inch ovenproof skillet over medium-high heat. Add the onion and cook, stirring, until soft, about 10 minutes.

- Add the spinach and tomatoes and cook, stirring, until wilted, about 5 minutes.

- Pour the egg mixture over the vegetable mixture and sprinkle with cheese. Transfer the skillet to the oven and bake until set about 15 minutes.

- Cut into wedges and serve with whole-wheat toast or a green salad if desired.

Nutritional value (per serving):

- Calories: 215

- Fat: 13 g

- Carbohydrates: 9 g

- Fiber: 2 g

- Protein: 16 g

Cooking time: 35 minutes

9. Lentil and Vegetable Stew

Ingredients:

- 1 tablespoon canola oil

- 1 onion, chopped

- 2 carrots, chopped

- 2 celery stalks, chopped

- 2 cloves garlic, minced

- 4 cups low sodium vegetable broth

- 2 cups water

- 1 (14.5-ounce) can diced tomatoes

- 1 cup brown lentils, rinsed and drained

- 2 teaspoons dried thyme

- 1/4 teaspoon salt

- 1/4 teaspoon black pepper

- 2 cups chopped kale

Preparation:

- Heat the oil in a large pot over medium-high heat. Add the onion, carrots, celery, and garlic and cook, stirring, until soft, about 10 minutes.

- Add the broth, water, tomatoes, lentils, thyme, salt, and pepper, and bring to a boil. Reduce the heat and simmer, covered, until the lentils are tender about 30 minutes.

- Stir in the kale and cook until wilted about 5 minutes. Serve with crusty bread or crackers if desired.

Nutritional value (per serving):

- Calories: 228

- Fat: 4 g

- Carbohydrates: 38 g

- Fiber: 16 g

- Protein: 13 g

Cooking time: 50 minutes

10. Turkey and Vegetable Sloppy Joes

Ingredients:

- 1 tablespoon canola oil

- 1 pound lean ground turkey

- 1 onion, chopped

- 1 green bell pepper, chopped

- 2 cloves garlic, minced

- 1 (15-ounce) can tomato sauce

- 1/4 cup ketchup

- 2 tablespoons Worcestershire sauce

- 1 tablespoon brown sugar

- 1 teaspoon chili powder

- 1/4 teaspoon salt

- 1/4 teaspoon black pepper

- 8 whole-wheat hamburger buns

- 8 lettuce leaves

- 8 slices tomato

Preparation:

- Heat the oil in a large skillet over medium-high heat. Add the turkey and cook, breaking it up with a wooden spoon, until browned and cooked through, about 10 minutes. Transfer to a plate and keep warm.

- In the same skillet, add the onion, bell pepper, and garlic and cook, stirring, until soft, about 10 minutes.

- Stir in the tomato sauce, ketchup, Worcestershire sauce, brown sugar, chili powder, salt and pepper and bring to a boil. Reduce the heat and simmer, uncovered, until slightly thickened, about 15 minutes.

- Return the turkey to the skillet and stir to combine. Spoon the mixture over the bottom halves of the buns and top with lettuce, tomato, and the top halves of the buns. Serve with baked fries or coleslaw if desired.

Nutritional value (per serving):

- Calories: 295

- Fat: 9 g

- Carbohydrates: 36 g

- Fiber: 6 g

- Protein: 21 g

Cooking time: 40 minutes

Chapter 7

Special Considerations
Nutrition and Exercise for Different Body Types

Have you ever pondered why some people manage to lose weight quickly while others find it difficult to reduce their body weight? One explanation could be because various body types have unique metabolic and hormonal traits that influence how they react to exercise and nutrition. The ectomorph, mesomorph, and endomorph are the three primary body types identified by the body type hypothesis. For the best results in weight loss, each body type has unique strengths and weaknesses that may necessitate varying activity and nutrition regimens. A synopsis of each body type is provided below, along with some advice on diet and exercise regimens for weight loss.

Ectomorph: Ectomorphs have a quick metabolism, a low body fat percentage, and are usually long-limbed, slender, and lean. They may also struggle to put on muscle and strength, even though they can consume a lot without gaining much weight. An ectomorph's diet should be high in calories, high in carbohydrates, and moderate in protein to give them the energy and nutrients they need to maintain their activity and muscular building.

A moderate-intensity, high-volume, low-frequency workout regimen that emphasizes resistance training and complex movements may also be beneficial for them in order to stimulate their muscle fibers and build more bulk and strength in their muscles.

Mesomorph: A mesomorph has a balanced metabolism, a moderate level of body fat, and is usually muscular, athletic, and well-proportioned. They can swiftly grow muscle and strength and, depending on their diet and exercise habits, gain or lose weight with ease. In order to maintain their weight and muscle mass without experiencing excessive weight gain or loss, mesomorphs may benefit from eating a diet that is balanced, diverse, and moderately caloric. To increase their muscular and cardiovascular fitness as well as their body composition, they might also benefit from a high-intensity, moderate-volume, moderate-frequency exercise program that combines resistance and cardio training.

Endomorph: Having a slow metabolism and a high percentage of body fat, endomorphs are usually rounded, soft, and curvaceous. Not only do they frequently put on weight, particularly in the lower body, but they may also struggle to shed fat and lose weight. A diet low in calories, low in carbohydrates, and high in protein may be beneficial for endomorphs in order to produce a calorie deficit, lower blood sugar and insulin levels, and encourage fat burning rather than fat storage. In order to boost their calorie expenditure and fat oxidation as well as their endurance and metabolism, they might also benefit from a low-intensity, high-frequency, high-duration exercise program that focuses on cardio and circuit training.

Weight Loss for Specific Health Conditions

Numerous medical disorders, including diabetes, high blood pressure, high cholesterol, heart disease, stroke, osteoarthritis, and certain malignancies, can benefit from weight loss. However, some persons with certain medical conditions, such as eating disorders, kidney illness, liver disease, thyroid abnormalities, or eating disorders, may find it difficult or dangerous to lose weight. As a result, it's crucial to speak with your doctor before beginning any weight loss program and to stick to a customized schedule that fits your requirements and preferences. Some broad pointers and recommendations for losing weight in relation to particular medical conditions:

- Diabetes: This illness affects the way your body uses glucose, a form of sugar that serves as your cells' primary energy source. Diabetes is characterized by either an excess or a shortage of glucose in the blood, which can lead to a number of problems, including heart disease, kidney damage, nerve damage, and eye damage.

Losing weight can help diabetics better control their blood pressure, cholesterol, and blood sugar levels as well as lessen their risk of problems. Nevertheless, medication dose, blood glucose levels, and hunger can all be impacted by weight loss. As a result, diabetics should eat a balanced diet that is high in fiber, low in carbohydrates, and moderate in protein. They should also routinely check their blood glucose levels. They should also exercise on a regular basis, but they shouldn't work out if their blood sugar is too high or too low, or if they exhibit any symptoms of complications, such ulcers on their feet or issues with their eyes.

- High blood pressure: Also known as hypertension, high blood pressure is a condition that can harm your heart, brain, kidneys, eyes, and other organs as well as your blood vessels when there is an excessive force of blood against the walls of your arteries. People with high blood pressure who lose weight can lower their blood pressure and lower their chance of developing heart disease, stroke, and renal disease. But losing weight can also have an impact on their fluid balance, salt sensitivity, and medicine dosage. As a result, individuals with high blood pressure should limit their intake of alcohol and caffeine and stick to a low-salt, low-fat, high-potassium, and high-calcium diet. They should also exercise on a regular basis, but refrain from doing so if their blood pressure is abnormally high or low, or if they exhibit any symptoms of problems, such dizziness, shortness of breath, or chest pain.

- High cholesterol: Also known as hyperlipidemia, this disorder is brought on by an excess of the fat type cholesterol in the blood. This fat can clog your arteries and produce blockages, which can result in peripheral artery disease, heart disease, or stroke. People with high cholesterol can lower their cholesterol and lower their risk of cardiovascular events by losing weight. However, their lipid profile, inflammation, and medicine dose may all be impacted by weight loss. As a result, those who have high cholesterol should reduce their intake of red meat, eggs, dairy, and processed foods and adopt a low-fat, low-saturated-fat, low-cholesterol, high-fiber, and high-omega-3 diet. They should also exercise on a regular basis, but they shouldn't work out if their cholesterol is too high or too low, or if they exhibit any symptoms of problems, including numbness, leg discomfort, or chest pain.

Nutritional Supplements and Their Role

Supplemental nutrition products are made with vitamins, minerals, herbs, or other ingredients to enhance the diet and improve health. In an attempt to speed up their metabolism, decrease hunger, or prevent the absorption of fat or carbohydrates, some people utilize nutritional supplements to help them lose weight. These supplements shouldn't be used in place of a healthy diet and regular exercise, though, as their efficacy and safety are frequently questioned.

Numerous nutritional supplement varieties make the claim to aid in weight loss; however, their modes of action and efficacy vary. Here are a few of the more typical ones:

- Caffeine: A stimulant, caffeine can make you burn more calories, enhance thermogenesis, burn fat, and feel less tired and hungry. Energy drinks, tea, coffee, and certain supplements all contain caffeine. However, there are other negative effects of caffeine that include jitteriness, anxiety, sleeplessness, and elevated blood pressure and heart rate. It's uncertain what the ideal caffeine dosage is for weight loss, however it can vary based on tolerance and sensitivity.

- Green tea extract: Packed with antioxidant and anti-inflammatory qualities, catechins are a kind of polyphenol found in green tea extract. Additionally, when taken with caffeine, catechins can increase fat oxidation and thermogenesis. Powders, capsules, and tea are all forms of green tea extract. On the other hand, adverse reactions including diarrhea, vomiting, nausea, and liver damage can also result from green tea extract. Although the exact amount and kind of catechins and caffeine in the extract may influence the best dosage for weight loss, this is not known.

- Garcinia cambogia: This tropical fruit has hydroxy citric acid (HCA), which can block the enzyme that turns carbohydrates into fat and raise serotonin levels, which are brain chemicals that control mood and hunger. Liquids, pills, and capsules are available forms of Garcinia Cambogia. On the other hand, garcinia cambogia may also result in adverse symptoms like headache, lightheadedness, dry mouth, and stomach pain. Although it's unknown exactly how much garcinia cambogia is best for weight loss, the recommended daily amount is between 500 and 1500 mg of HCA.

- Raspberry ketones: These are the molecules that give raspberries their flavor and scent. Adiponectin, a hormone that controls glucose and fat metabolism, can also be increased, as can the breakdown and release of fat from fat cells. Raspberry ketones are available as liquids, pills, or capsules. On the other hand, jitteriness, palpitations, and elevated blood pressure are some of the adverse consequences of raspberry ketones. Although the ideal dosage of raspberry ketones for weight loss is unknown, it may be as little as 100–200 mg daily.

Chapter 8

Lifestyle Changes for Long-Term Success

Building Sustainable Habits

Developing permanent weight reduction habits doesn't mean sticking to a rigid diet or exercise schedule; instead, it means adopting gradual, consistent changes that suit your tastes and way of life. Long-term routines that you can stick with without experiencing deprivation, boredom, or tension are known as sustainable habits. The following advice and actions will help you create long-lasting weight loss habits:

- Determine your motivation and objectives: You must decide why you want to lose weight and what your objectives are before you can begin your weight loss journey. Instead, then being driven by pressure from the outside world or irrational expectations, your motivation and goals should be deeply personal and significant to you. For instance, you might wish to reduce weight in order to enjoy a particular activity or occasion, or to enhance your performance, confidence, or health. To help you remember your direction and purpose, put your motivation and goals in writing and refer to them frequently.

- Start by changing one habit at a time. Attempting to modify too many habits at once can be stressful and ineffective. Instead, concentrate on one habit at a time, and simplify and ease the process as much as you can. For instance, you could begin by increasing your water intake, vegetable intake, or walking frequency. You can progressively develop your healthy lifestyle by starting with one habit and working your way up to another.

- help it pleasurable and rewarding: Encouraging and rewarding behaviors will help you look forward to completing them and feel good about yourself, which is one of the cornerstones to developing durable habits. For instance, you can work out while engaging in an activity you enjoy, like dancing, swimming, or playing sports, or you can work out while listening to music, podcasts, or audiobooks. In addition, you can treat yourself to something that will help you reach your weight loss objectives, like massage, book, or new clothes. You can also celebrate your accomplishments with loved ones, friends, or on social media.

Follow your progress and modify your strategy: Monitoring your progress and making necessary adjustments to your plan is another essential component of developing long-lasting habits. You can monitor your progress using a variety of instruments and techniques, including a notebook, a calendar, an app, a scale, a tape measure, or a picture.

You can see how far you have come, what works and what doesn't, as well as the chances and challenges you face, by keeping track of your progress. Additionally, based on your outcomes and feedback, you may use your progress to modify your plan. For example, you can add or remove a habit or change your intensity, frequency, or duration.

- Have forgiveness and patience: It takes time and work to create long-lasting weight loss habits, and obstacles and failures are commonplace along the route. Be nice and compassionate to yourself; instead of being harsh or giving up on yourself, practice patience and forgiveness. Keep in mind that every day is an opportunity to start over and that every step matters. You can also ask for assistance and motivation from those who can keep you on course and get beyond any obstacles.

Incorporating Physical Activity into Daily Life

Any weight loss plan should include physical activity because it can help you burn calories, enhance your mood, and improve your health. However, many people find it difficult to find the time and motivation to exercise, particularly if they have hectic schedules, little money, or inadequate levels of fitness. Thankfully, there are lots of ways to fit exercise into your daily schedule without having to purchase pricey equipment, sign up for a gym membership, or adhere to a rigid schedule. Here are some pointers and illustrations on how to do that:

- Make it a habit: One of the most important things to accomplish when integrating physical activity into your daily routine is to make it a habit—that is, something you do on a regular basis without giving it any thought. Selecting an activity that you enjoy, fits into your lifestyle and tastes, and is easy and consistent to perform is essential to forming a habit. It is imperative that you establish a precise time and location for your task and associate it with an ingrained routine or cue, such finishing your morning meal, brushing your teeth, or quitting work. For instance, you may choose to always use the stairs rather than the elevator when you enter or exit a building, or you could opt to walk for fifteen minutes first thing every morning.

- Make it enjoyable and social: Including physical activity in your everyday routine can also be accomplished by making it enjoyable and social, something you look forward to and that makes you happy. To achieve this, pick an activity that brings you joy, challenge, or satisfaction, like dancing, playing sports, or gardening. Involving those who can encourage, support, and keep you accountable—like your family, friends, coworkers, or neighbors—is another way to achieve this.

For instance, you may arrange a friendly soccer match with your coworkers, enroll in a dancing class, or join a neighborhood walking group.

- Make it convenient and accessible: This is a third strategy for incorporating physical activity into your daily routine. It should be something you can do whenever and wherever you choose, without requiring a lot of time, money, or effort. You can accomplish this by selecting a physical activity, like walking, jogging, or skipping, that doesn't call for specialized tools, spaces, or knowledge. Using the resources and opportunities found in your immediate surroundings, such as parks, trails, walkways, and stairs, is another way you can accomplish this. For instance, you can park your car further away from your destination, walk or ride your bike to work or school, or use your lunch break to perform some squats or stretches.

Maintaining Weight Loss Maintenance

It might be difficult to sustain a weight loss after it has been lost. Many people who lose weight find that they gain it back within a few years or even months because of a variety of circumstances, including hormone fluctuations, lifestyle changes, metabolic slowdown, and psychological issues. However, with the right techniques and assistance, maintaining a weight loss is achievable. The following are some pointers and actions to keep up weight loss:

- Maintain a balanced and flexible diet: Eating a balanced and flexible diet that meets your needs for calories and nutrients without being overly restrictive or monotonous is one of the secrets to keeping off the weight. Variety from several food groups, such as fruits, vegetables, whole grains, lean proteins, healthy fats, and low-fat dairy, should be a part of a balanced diet. Foods heavy in calories, fat, sugar, and salt, such as processed, fried, or fast food, should be avoided. With a flexible diet, you should be able to modify your consumption based on your tastes, activity level, and level of hunger while still occasionally enjoying your favorite foods without feeling restricted or guilty. Additionally, you can measure your food and nutrient intake with a food journal, tracker, or app to observe how it affects your ability to maintain your weight.

- Continue your physical activity: Staying physically active can help you burn calories, preserve your muscle mass, increase your metabolism, and enhance your overall health and fitness. It is also essential for maintaining weight loss. Any kind of action that causes you to perspire and elevate your heart rate, such as cycling, swimming, dancing, or jogging, is considered physical activity. Strength training is another option; it can improve your body composition and help you gain and maintain muscle mass and strength. It is generally advised to perform strength training twice a week in addition to 150 minutes of moderate-to-intense or 75 minutes of high-intensity exercise per week, or a mix of the two.

Additionally, you can track your physical activity and calorie expenditure with a fitness tracker, watch, or app to see how they impact your ability to maintain your weight.

- Track your weight and progress: Depending on your objectives and preferences, tracking your weight and progress on a frequent basis—ideally once a week or once a month—is essential to maintaining weight reduction. You can see how far you have come, what works and what doesn't, as well as what chances and obstacles you encounter, by keeping track of your weight and progress. A scale, a tape measure, an image, or a notebook are just a few of the instruments and techniques you might use to keep track of your weight and progress. A weight loss chart is another useful tool for tracking your progress and observing how your diet and level of physical activity relate to your weight. A weight loss calculator can also be used to determine your target weight and body fat percentage, as well as your caloric and nutritional requirements, based on your age, gender, height, weight, degree of exercise, and weight reduction objective.

- Seek help and input: Getting support and feedback from people who can motivate, inspire, and hold you accountable for your weight maintenance is a fourth key to keeping weight off. You can ask your family, friends, coworkers, or neighbors for support and input.

They can hear about your struggles, triumphs, and experiences and can also provide you with resources, guidance, and tips. Professionals who can offer you expert coaching, monitoring, and evaluation include your doctor, a nutritionist, or a personal trainer. You may also ask for support and comments from these individuals. You can also interact with people who share your interests and goals by joining a fitness class, weight loss club, or online community. Here, you can share ideas, support, and information with like-minded individuals.

Conclusion

Weight loss is a common and desirable goal for many people, as it can improve their health, appearance, and well-being. However, weight loss is not a simple or easy process, and it requires a comprehensive and personalized approach that involves nutrition, exercise, and lifestyle changes. In this book, we have discussed the various aspects of nutrition and exercise for weight loss and provided you with evidence-based information, tips, and strategies to help you achieve your weight loss goals and maintain your results in the long term.

We have covered the following topics in this book:

- The basics of weight loss, such as the causes and consequences of excess weight, the factors that influence weight loss, and the methods and tools to measure and monitor weight loss.

- The role of nutrition for weight loss, such as the types and amounts of calories, macronutrients, and micronutrients that are needed for weight loss, the effects of different diets and dietary patterns on weight loss, and the strategies and habits to improve your nutrition and eating behavior for weight loss.

- The role of exercise for weight loss, such as the types and amounts of physical activity that are needed for weight loss, the effects of different exercises and exercise modes on weight loss, and the strategies and habits to improve your physical activity and exercise performance for weight loss.

- The role of lifestyle for weight loss, such as the effects of sleep, stress, and mental health on weight loss, and the strategies and habits to improve your sleep, stress, and mental health for weight loss.

- The challenges and solutions for weight loss, such as the common barriers and obstacles that can hinder your weight loss progress, and the solutions and resources that can help you overcome them and stay on track with your weight loss plan.

- The maintenance and prevention of weight regain, such as the factors and mechanisms that can cause weight regain after weight loss, and the strategies and habits to prevent and manage weight regain and maintain your weight loss results.

We hope that this book has provided you with valuable and practical information, tips, and strategies to help you lose weight and keep it off for life. We also hope that this book has inspired you to adopt a healthy and balanced lifestyle that suits your needs and preferences and that you enjoy and can sustain for life. Remember, weight loss is a personal and gradual process, and you should be patient, consistent, and supportive of yourself along the way. You can also seek support and feedback from others who can encourage you, inspire you, and hold you accountable for your weight loss goals.

We wish you all the best in your weight loss journey, and we look forward to hearing about your success stories. Thank you for reading this book.

www.ingramcontent.com/pod-product-compliance
Lightning Source LLC
Chambersburg PA
CBHW070808260726

48660CB00005B/1772